Running

Running for Beginners: A comprehensive guide on how to get started on the road to a fitter you!

By

Faye Froome

Faye Froome Copyright © 2016

Disclaimer

No part of this publication may be reproduced or transmitted in any form or by any means, mechanical or electronic, including photocopying or recording, or by any information storage and retrieval system, or transmitted by email without permission in writing from the publisher.

While all attempts and efforts have been made to verify the information held within this publication, neither the author nor the publisher assumes any responsibility for errors, omissions, or opposing interpretations of the content herein.

This book is for entertainment purposes only. The views expressed are those of the author alone, and should not be taken as expert instruction or commands. The reader of this book is responsible for his or her own actions when it comes to reading the book.

Adherence to all applicable laws and regulations, including international, federal, state, and local governing professional licensing, business practices, advertising, and all other aspects of doing business in the US, Canada, or any other jurisdiction is the sole responsibility of the purchaser or reader.

Neither the author nor the publisher assumes any responsibility or liability whatsoever on the behalf of the purchaser or reader of these materials.

Any received slight of any individual or organization is purely unintentional.

Table of Contents

Introduction

Running is one of the best ways to train for fitness, lose weight and improve your health through exercise. In spite of this many people struggle to develop a running hobby for a myriad of reasons, including purchasing the incorrect gear or using a poor running technique.

This down-to-earth and straight-forward guide will provide you with all the information you will need to grow and flourish as a runner, becoming healthier and happier in the process.

In the first chapter you will learn about the proper gear to buy, including learning how to buy the correct shoes, socks and even accessories such as lubricant. You will also learn how to take care of your feet and avoid injuries. The second chapter will cover you through the topics of nutrition and weight loss, helping you understand the importance of diet and how to correctly make a post-workout meal.

Meanwhile the third chapter will cover proper running technique and form, covering details such as pronation and running up and down hills as well as pacing.

The fourth chapter will help you work on your mentality and mental fortitude, whilst the fifth chapter will tackle various health and safety concerns such as staying visible, avoiding danger and managing hay fever and asthma that can often cause novice runners to quit during the summer months. Let's get going!

Chapter 1 – Running Gear

Equipment & Foot Care

When starting running as a hobby it is important to invest in a high quality pair of shoes that matches your individual needs. Generally speaking, when people run their feet can land in one of three ways; a neutral position, an over-pronation position or a supination position. A neutral position is the best, resulting in less chance of injury to the feet, ankles and legs and allows for a greater variety of show choices.

However, if you have a tendency to pronate or supinate when you run, this often cannot be helped. Pronation is the habit of rolling your foot inwards as you make contact with the ground. When we walk or run our foot needs to pronate to absorb the shock and impact from the collision between our foot and the floor.

Nonetheless many people do not pronate properly, either failing to mitigate the shock properly or exaggerate the movement too much, placing stress on their joints, tendons and muscles. Over-pronation is when the foot rolls inward too much, where as supination, also known as under-pronation, is the habit of rolling the foot outward.

Depending on whether your foot lands in a neutral position, an over-pronation position or a supination position will influence what shoes are ideal for you. If you over-pronate or supinate you will need corrective shoes that counteract your bad habit. For over-pronators you will want motion control shoes whereas for supinators you will want stability shoes. People who pronate correctly can wear regular running shoes, but also shoes with neutral cushioning or lightweight variants.

Most good running or sport stores will offer advice and guidance on the type of pronation you have and will be able to offer you the correct running shoes to purchase. Many stores will be able to test you on their running machines completely free of charge.

You will need to replace your running shoes occasionally as once they become worn; they will influence your pronation habits and may increase the chance of injury. Typically it is recommended that you replace your running shoes between every 350-500 miles. Of course this is a loose estimate and you should always apply common sense when thinking about whether you need a new pair of shoes.

A simple test to determine whether your shoes are becoming worn is to place them on a completely flat surface and see whether they tilt – if they tilt in one particular direction that suggests one side of the shoe has become worn.

You should also make an effort to maintain your shoes whilst you use them. After running in wet conditions it can be tempting to place your shoes against a radiator or in a warm place to help the dry. However doing this will cause your shoes to shrink over time, which can result in blisters and other foot problems. Likewise if you keep your shoes in a cold area, such as an outside porch, they will contract which will damage the cushioning and support build into the shoe.

The best solution is to allow your shoes to dry naturally in a dry place and invest in multiple pairs of shoes if your shoes do not dry enough between runs.

In terms of fit, running shoes with laces typically fit better and should be preferred if you are prone to blisters or have an unusual foot shape and struggle to find shoes that suit you. If you find that your joints or tendons are hurting after frequent runs you should favor rubber-soled shoes with generous amounts of cushioning which will help you absorb impact against the ground better. If the sole of your cushioned shoes feels hard after prolonged use, this is a good indicator that it might be time to buy a new pair of shoes.

When purchasing a pair of running shoes, wear the running socks you intend to wear with them. Socks will alter how the shoe fits and feels, so wearing socks that you won't pair with those shoes might give you a bad impression of the fit. Generally speaking for running enthusiasts it is best to go a specialized running shoe store that will have members of staff trained to look at how you walk and run and the shape of your feet and then recommend a type of shoe.

In addition to shoes you should also invest in several pair of running socks. A well-fitting pair of running socks will prevent you from getting blisters; however socks also form an important role in keeping your feet dry. In particular avoid wearing cotton socks which are prone to making your feet wet and forming blisters. There are numerous different thicknesses and alternate materials available so it is best just to buy several different pairs and see which ones work for you.

Blisters can also be avoided through the use of a lubricant applied to the feet and the outside of the socks before running. Lubricants reduce the friction between your skin, the socks and the shoes, therefore reducing the overall amount of rubbing and irritation. Applying lubricant in this way had the added benefit of also keeping your feet dry, which can be useful on wet days. Vaseline works great as a lubricant but most types of petroleum jelly will also work fine.

Lubricants can also help prevent chaffing, so for especially long runs or for larger runners applying a little lubricant to the thighs and the armpits can be beneficial. Some male runners wearing loose tops and running great distances actually report chaffing against the nipples – which can also be avoided with a little grease if you are unfortunate to suffer with this problem. For people who really struggle with chaffing, applying grease to the inside of the clothes can also help.

If you're prone to dry feet, it can be useful to frequently moisturize your feet to prevent large skin cracks from occurring which will put a stop to your running habits for at least several days. There are hundreds of different brands available – the more important factor is the method of application. Moisturize your feet after a bath and shower whilst the skin is still tender. Rub the entirety of the feet with the moisturizer until the feet have become soft and smooth to the touch.

Of course you also need to make an effort to avoid your feet from getting too wet, which is the biggest factor in causing an Athlete's foot infection. You can keep your feet dry by allowing your shoes to dry between runs, avoiding running when the ground it too wet, never wearing the same pair of socks twice as well as investing in lightweight and waterproof socks and shoes if necessary. Some people also find it helpful to apply anti-perspirants to the feet to prevent them from sweating which is the predominant cause of moisture.

Athlete's foot is typically spread in locker rooms and gyms in which many people who rigorously exercise encounter each other and walk across the same floor. If you are especially worried about developing Athlete's foot you can wear flip flops or any light footwear in these public environments to limit the potential contact your foot has with the fungus in the area.
However, Athlete's foot can be dealt with using an over-the-counter medicine available from a local pharmacist if necessary. When using fungicide to deal with Athlete's foot it is particularly important to be consistent and disciplined with the application of your treatment as the fungus can develop a resistance to treatment and go into dormancy, only to return once you thought the problem was dealt with.

Some people may also experience swelling in their feet after they have run, due to various factors such as water movement, increased blood flow and overheating. The best solution to swelling is simply to apply cold water to your feet. For people who suffer from severe swelling you might want to purchase some Epsom salts which when added to water give it anti-swelling properties. However Epsom salts can cause your feet to become dry if used too much, so be careful.

Above and all other considerations the most important aspect to keeping your feet in good condition is realizing that prevention is better than cure and applying damage control the moment you notice a problem. It is easy to think you can simply 'man-up' over a small problem, but if you consistently run you are just going to make that blister, infection, swelling, etc worse. Instead of false bravado, deal with the problem at the source whilst it is still small and easily manageable. Better still, take steps to avoid getting a problem altogether through buying the right equipment and using preventative measures such as lubricant. Even though taking the initiative to prevent trouble requires a little upfront effort it will save you time and suffering in the long-term.

Finally you may also want to use specific exercise that trains your toes, feet, ankles and calves to be stronger. It takes a great deal of time for the muscles in these regions to grow enough to deal with running sizable distances multiple times in a week. You can speed up this process by selectively stressing these muscles and forcing them to grow faster. However be careful not to overdo it if your muscles are already aching. Even if you don't push your running limits, developing strong muscles in your legs and feet can change the way your feet move whilst running, reducing the chance of injury.

The simplest exercise to practice is calf raises, an exercise where you stand upright with your feet a few inches apart and push upwards with your toes. Hold this pose for a brief moment before relaxing steadily – repeat this motion 20-30 times to build up strength in your toes and calves. For people with stronger calves and toes, you may want to rest your toes on a raised surface, such as a small bench, to increase the resistance and effort required.

You can also stretch your toes directly by sitting on the floor with your legs stretched out in front of you and pulling on your toes with your hands (or a piece of cloth if you cannot reach).

Clothes

Selecting clothes to run in is much easier than selecting a pair of running shoes. Anything that is light and relatively loose is a good choice, as your main concern is having enough freedom to move and not increasing the amount of weight you have to run with.

Nonetheless as an aspiring running enthusiast you may want to purchase some speciality running clothes which are designed to have a few perks. For example, wicker t-shirts are a type of t-shirt made especially for runners which have the magical quality of moving sweat away from your skin and to the outside of the shirt, where it will evaporate quicker. This helps keep your drier and results in less soreness. Furthermore as the sweat evaporates, moisture doesn't weigh down the t-shirt, resulting in it being lighter.

If you are female, you will almost always want to invest in a sports-bra. Ligaments in the breast can stretch and tear whilst running, not only causing ache but also irreversible sag. Sports bras drastically reduce movement whilst you run, preventing damage and sag.

A good pair of shorts will generally suffice for clothing below the waist. If you find that your thighs chafe, your shorts may be too tight or be made of an unsuitable material, so considering sourcing a replacement.

For advanced runners, however, you might want to consider trying out a pair of running tights. Please be aware this is for both men and women! Tights can provide better warmth insulation, which is great for both winter and early morning running. However tights can also be made of wicking material and be made to be especially breathable, therefore helping you deal with sweat and airflow.

The design of running tights is also intended to help reduce chafe and irritation. Finally, tights offer a competitive edge. Tights improve how aerodynamic your legs are, which can improve your running speed and lower the amount of energy your runs require. Although it is not yet fully understood or supported, there are also small amounts of evidence to suggest that wearing tights can improve blood flow and increase the speed at which the muscles recover from exercise as a result. Therefore if you really want to take your running to the next level, tights can be essential.

If you want to keep your running practice going through winter, you are going to need to winter gear. Thermal vests and thermal underwear can help, but in most circumstances you are going to need to pay out for a running jacket which will keep you protected from the wind and cold. You will need to go to a speciality running or activity store to buy a suitable jacket as most outdoor jackets will be far too heavy and cumbersome to actually run in.

Furthermore when buying a running jacket favor bright and high visibility jackets that can help keep you safe during the evening when vehicles and pedestrians might not be able to see you. This can also apply to any wicking t-shirts you purchase.

To combat the cold you might also want to wear a simple of gloves and a beanie. Beanies are more aerodynamic than other choices such as caps and hoodies and they stay in place, even during windy days when other headwear does not.

Other Gear

Keeping a sport watch whilst you run is a great idea if you are concerned about the speed of your runs or you use time as a measurement of distance. Sports watches are generally a lighter than regular watches or a smart phone and come with specific setting for timing laps or routines. Advanced sport watches can also come with features such as calorie counters and even cross-device compatibility allowing you to upload data to a computer and track your performance in great detail. On a similar vein a heart rate monitor can also be useful. Above and beyond the fact that measuring your heart rate is kind of cool, knowing how hard your heart is working is a good metric to evaluate how much effort you are putting into your run.

Sometimes our mood or other circumstantial factors can influence how we feel when we are running and if we are pushing ourselves enough – it is easy to deceive yourself into believing that you are doing enough, or not realizing if you are going too far! A heart rate monitor gives you an objective and unbiased measurement of just how much stress your body is under – vital for performance based running.

Some runners like to carry a source of water around with them. Generally speaking unless you are doing a particularly long run (90 minutes or more) or unless the day is especially hot, carrying water with you is unnecessary for keeping safely hydrated, although it may help increase performance.

Nonetheless if you want to carry water around with you, there are several prominent choices. A donut shaped running water bottle will allow you to keep your water bottle easily in grip, which is great for shorter runs. For longer runs, or if you want to bring alongside a few extra accessories such as a phone or your keys, you can get a 'handheld bottle carrier' which has a fabric based bag attached to the water bottle where you can store your vitals.

For long-distance running that may take hours or even most of the day, taking a specially designed water pack with you, which functions like a light-weight backpack with straws and attachments to drink from can be helpful. However consider that for longer organized running events water is often provided at stations along the route, so taking a water pack is often only important for longer solitary runs.

In terms of pure performance consuming a sports drink is a better choice than pure water. Sports drinks contain sugar for energy to keep you going, but also electrolyte which increases the speed at which your body absorbs water (helping you to hydrate faster). However, obviously, if you are running as a weight-loss solution these drinks are often high in calories and should be avoided.

In regards to hydration in general, it is important to keep your water consumption in mind, but unless you are greatly concerned about performance, don't over think it either. As previously mentioned for runs that are shorter than 60-90 minutes, taking water or a form of hydration with you isn't necessary.

Furthermore drinking too much water during exercise can be dangerous and cause a condition caused water poisoning. Water poisoning occurs when an individual consumes huge amounts of water whilst their body is deprived of sodium and electrolytes which helps the body deal with said water (electrolytes and sodium are lost during exercise).

The take-home point here is that in situations where hydration might be a genuine concern, it is often better to favour a sports drink. Also, although sometimes thirst can be deceptively strong or weak, generally your own sense of thirst is your best guide to whether you need to drink water during exercise.

Treadmills & Running

There are some important differences between running over ground and running over treadmills that you need to appreciate. Firstly, running over a treadmill is much easier than running over ground. The movement of the belt on the treadmill makes it easier to move your legs forward, effectively reducing your calorie expenditure. Therefore most runners find that their performance is better on the treadmill when compared to the outside.

Running on the treadmill also doesn't cause your feet to harden and become more resilient, as the treadmill is specifically designed to accommodate the collision of your feet with the floor. As a result people who are used to running on treadmills may find that they struggle to run on the ground normally.

However the treadmill is often a better tool for practicing and training, allowing you to measure your performance and adjust speed and incline for better recovery levels. In particular the treadmill is fantastic for speed running and slowing down in cycles.

Chapter 2 – Nutrition & Weight Loss

Nutrition for running

Your nutrition should follow a standard diet rules – focus on whole grains, nuts, fruit, vegetables, low-fat dairy and lean meats. Of course this is an ideal that most of us will stray from, but providing your body an adequate supply of nutrition is necessary for energy and recovery.

When taking upon a dietary plan for running you don't need to enact a strict calorie-counting meal-plan (although this is not necessarily a bad thing). However keeping track of what you are eating in a looser sense by writing down what you are eating everyday whilst you eat it is a good idea. Most of us can be ignorant of what we actually consume, forgetting the little snacks and treats we consume every day. When tracking what you consume, remember to also include oils, calorific drinks and dressings which often contain large amounts of calories that we fail to take heed of.

When you are mindful of what you are actually consuming you can create the space to enjoy a treat every now and then, otherwise your cravings can build up and make you break your healthy habits.

In terms of more detailed eating habits for running, your running nutrition largely depends on the type of running you are working towards. A runner who focuses on sprinting and sport sprints need to consider their diet in a different way from someone who is working towards a half-marathon, who in turn should be different from people who run full marathons.

For long-distance runners, your focus should be on managing your stores of carbohydrates. Your body can only store so much carbohydrate in your system at once, some of which you will gain from digesting carbohydrates in your stomach but some of which will be stored in your muscles as a source of energy.

When your carbohydrate supply runs dry, your body will be forced to burn fat for energy. This sounds appealing, especially for people looking to lose weight, but it can lead to an energy 'wall' that is incredibly hard to push past. The current research suggests that your body will run out of carbohydrate stores around 2 hours into an intense workout, which is often notably before the end-goal in a marathon or similar length run.

Therefore you should look to eat meals high in carbohydrate before long-distance runs – whole grain bread, cereals, or grains are good choices. However, don't eat your meal immediately before you run. When you run your body diverts energy away from digestion and towards your muscles and your respiratory system. Therefore if you've eaten a large meal just before a run it won't be digested in time and it might uncomfortably bounce in your stomach. Allow yourself at least a 1-2 hour window between eating a meal and running any length of distance. Generally speaking, the closer to your run the lighter your meal should be – you don't want your stomach to be full during your run.

There is some evidence that for novice runners whose glycogen stores are not as well developed as better-trained runners that running in a carbohydrate deprived state can help them develop better glycogen stores in the future. Nonetheless, for experienced runners you should always ensure an adequate carbohydrate supply to avoid an energy deficit.

When you feel that you hit that energy wall then you should start to consume glucose drinks to allow you to refresh your stores of carbohydrate and maintain your pace.

Post-workout is an entirely different story. Post-workout your focus should be primarily consuming proteins to allow your muscles to rebuild any damage they sustain during your session. You should also consume a light snack so your muscles can build up a store of glycogen – the carbohydrate stored in your muscles – otherwise you might feel a distinct lag and energy deficit in a few hours.

For faster runs and sprints your dietary focus is different. You want to eat carbs before your sprints, but the carbs you want to eat should be easily digestible and rapidly absorbed rather than complex carbohydrates that are broken down over the course of an hour or so. Evidence suggests that within the 30 minutes of recovery there is a window where nutrients are absorbed quicker and more efficiently, but only for relatively intense workouts. Intense workouts should be understood as relative to your usual level of activity – that might be a few hours for a trained runner, but 30 minutes for a complete novice.

Furthermore, post-workout for speed running, you want to eat more or less immediately. It is recommended that you eat in a proportion of roughly 4: 1 of carbohydrates to proteins, with a particularly good and tasty source being chocolate milk, which matches these proportions. In fact several studies suggest that chocolate milk outperforms most post-workout drinks manufactured to help improve recovery and helping yourself to a little treat can lighten the mood when your exercise starts to feel less rewarding. Other good choices include a banana with two tablespoons of peanut butter, half a cup of natural yogurt with some fruit or a fried egg with a little spinach.

Although it might seem best to consume a higher amount of protein, your body needs the carbohydrates to help break down the protein quicker and absorb these nutrients within the recovery window. Higher levels of protein actually limit digestion, resulting in less protein absorbed by the body within a short time frame.

Some people find that they have an unsettled stomach after running and that they struggle to eat food for a few hours. Eating food in the correct carbohydrate to protein ratio will be beneficial but you can also try having a smoothie or a shake instead, as liquid food will be easier to tolerate.

There is also a recovery window between 1-3 hours after your session. During this recovery window your nutrition should be slightly different – you should favor a higher protein meal which also includes a healthy fat, such as olive oil or avocados, whilst cutting down a little of the carbohydrates. Good suggestions for this meal include a salad with grilled chicken, a vegetable omelet with a piece of fruit or a serving of chili.

The number of calories you will burn will depend upon your mass and the intensity of your workout, although for most people of an average weight 100 calories per mile is a good estimation of how much energy you will burn. The intention in terms of calories should be to eat only what your body needs to recover, neither depriving yourself nor gorging yourself.

Of course if you are running to lose weight you may go without a post-workout meal, but you should expect this to influence both your performance and your recovery time for future sessions.

Therefore you need to plan to get an adequate calorie count, as if you burn too many calories you might end up losing muscle mass or recovering too slowly from your sessions.

There is some research to suggest that consuming caffeine is beneficial to runners, as studies have reported that runners who drink coffee or another caffeinated drink generally receive better 5k running times, perform better in higher temperatures, increasing power and speed and help your body metabolize and burn fat. There is some concern that as caffeine is a diuretic – a substance that helps you lose water – that is might have an adverse effect on performance during elongated runs, however the research literature suggests that mild to moderate caffeine consumption doesn't impact water loss during exercise.

The ideal level of caffeine consumption was found to be around 5mg per lb of bodyweight, which amounts to a large cup of filtered coffee for an average weight person, although this will obviously depend upon the brand of coffee you use. Caffeine lasts in the body for several hours whilst also being consumed quickly, which makes caffeine a good choice for consumption immediately before a run but also during your meal earlier in the day.

With that being established, it is best to experiment and find what works for you. It is especially important to be familiar with the effects before you start changing your diet – drinking a huge cup of coffee before a marathon for example might improve performance, but it might just make your body go haywire. It's best just to play it safe.

Weight Loss

If you are running for weight loss you should employ different dietary principles. The important aspect about losing weight and retaining performance is that you need to be informed about what is the correct weight for your body. It is better to think less in terms of weight and more about body composition. If you have more muscle or you are taller than your peers then weighing more is natural and you shouldn't force yourself to try and reach a designated weight just for the sake of it.

Your percentage body fat is usually a better indication of your health and whether you should be looking to gain or lose weight. For men a health body fat percentage is between 5-15%, with the lower spectrum being more specifically aimed towards athletes and bodybuilders. For women, who naturally have a higher percentage of body fat and less muscle, a range between 7 -28% is healthy, again with the lower spectrum being more towards professional athletes and people who train intensively.

It is relatively popular in recent years to cut carbohydrates in order to lose weight in a variation of a ketogenic diet, which forces your body to burn fat or protein. Nonetheless as running depends on glycogen and carbohydrate burning this will notably impair your performance and make it harder to run. If you are using running as your primary method of exercise and weight loss, do not cut carbohydrates!

Also bear in mind that you might gain weight whilst running because you gain muscle. This is not a bad thing! As mentioned earlier you should be more concerned about your body composition rather than your weight value. Muscle actually weighs more than fat in terms of the space it requires on your body as muscle is denser than fat. As a result even if you lose substantial levels of fat, muscle gain can actually counteract this in terms of weight quite easily. Overall, if you don't have an easy method to measure your body composition than use how you feel, how you look and how your clothes feel as indicators of whether running is being successful for you.

Another factor you need to consider is the weight of your glycogen reserves. For new runners, there glycogen reserves can increase up to 70% over the first few months of endurance running. It is thought that for every 1oz of glycogen your body stores, it also retains 3oz of water. As water is obviously heavy, this might lead to a misleading number of the scale.

The final piece of advice is that you shouldn't use running as an excuse to increase the amount that you eat. This sounds obvious but for endurance runners it is often all too true that we gorge ourselves after a gruesome run because we feel like we deserve it or we somehow believe that a faster metabolism will make everything alright. Worthiness or metabolism magic aside, calories are calories and if you consume more calories than you expend you will not lose weight.

Therefore try to stick to the post-workout nutrition recommended in this guide. As mentioned earlier, 100 calories per mile is a good rough estimate of your calorie expenditure, with that figure being slightly less for slower and lighter runners and slightly more for heavier and faster runners. Therefore if you just ran a 5 mile run, you've built a 500 calorie deficit. If you've only run 3 miles that a 300 calorie deficit, which will be more or less consumed by an overzealous post-workout snack.

As a side note, your body is manipulative. If you attempt to deny it energy after a run, it will produce cravings that will make sugary and fatty foods more attractive. The harder you try and deny yourself, the stronger these cravings will be. Therefore it isn't just about what you eat, but how fast you eat it – satiating these energy demands earlier will generally cause less temptation and influence to consume junk food later on in the day.

Cross Training

There is often a great deal of confusion about what cross-training is and how it relates to running. Cross-training is the practice of incorporating numerous different athletic training exercises into one program or regime. Cross-training is useful as different exercises work on different muscles resulting in a balanced and well-rounded practice.

In particular cross-training can help you develop stamina, which is a different concept to fitness. Fitness, or more specifically, cardiovascular fitness, the type of fitness involved in running, is the ability of the body to absorb and distribute oxygen around your body during exercise. Running is a fantastic way to build up cardiovascular fitness and long-distances runners will often have the best cardiovascular fitness out of any group of athletes.

Stamina or endurance is a more nuanced concept however. Stamina refers to your body's ability to sustain prolonged effort and exertion, which involves more than just oxygen supply and often relates to the strength and condition of the muscles. Undoubtedly there is a small overlap between these two concepts, yet nonetheless they remain their own distinct entities. Therefore it is possible to have high levels of stamina with low levels of fitness and high levels of fitness but with low levels of endurance.

The relevant point here is that running requires fitness but also endurance. However your endurance when running is often dependent on muscles that you may not be building when running itself. A powerful core and back helps maintain posture that can make your running more efficient and less tiresome whilst strong, resilient legs are needed to keep speed steady over longer distances.

Cross-training allows you to remedy this by building muscle and strength in ways that normal running wouldn't. Therefore if you want to make running more successful, try another sports such as swimming or weight lifting.

Chapter 3 – Running Form & Technique

Warming Up For a Run

It's important to warm-up and cool-down before and after a running session. Warming-up loosens your muscles and increases blood flow to your muscles, preparing them for intense periods of activity. For running the best warm-up activity is generally walking, which uses all the same muscles in more or less the exact same way. A 3-5 minute period of walking is a great way to start your warm up, but you should progress to a gentle jog and gentle stride before you finally commit to your run.

In terms of stretching a lot of the advice available is misinformed. An intense bout of stretching before running has actually been linked to greater risk of injury. Whilst stretching improves the condition of muscles, joint and tendons in the long-term, in the short-term it stresses them and makes them weaker.

However that doesn't mean you need to abandon stretching altogether. Rather you should switch from static stretching to dynamic stretching. Static stretching is the type of stretches where you hold a position for several moments, whilst dynamic stretching are flowing movements that loosen the muscles.

For example the hip flexor stretch is a simple dynamic stretch where the knee is raised towards the neck until the thigh is at a right angle towards the floor and the calf points down. It is hardly an exerting stretch, yet it nonetheless loosens the muscles in the leg and hips.

The leg extensor stretch is a similar dynamic stretch, bringing the foot up towards the buttocks, bending the leg at the knee. This stretch also helps improve your balance.

The planar flexor stretch involves keeping the leg straight and raising above the ground then bending the foot upwards at the ankle. Keeping your arms held around the waist can help you maintain balance whilst you flex.

The hip extensor stretch is a slightly more advanced dynamic stretch. In this stretch the back is bent forward and the leg is raised with the knee pointing forward and the calf facing the floor. Whilst leaning forward bring the raised leg behind the body.

There are many more simple dynamic stretches that can be practiced.

Running Technique

In addition to pronating correctly there are numerous aspects of running technique that you can practice to help improve your sessions.

The first is to focus on stride frequency rather than stride length. For runners, the speed of their run is determined by the length of your running stride multiplied by the frequency of your strides. To improve running speed it's better to focus on the number of strides rather than the length of the stride, at least as a beginner.

Taking longer strides is harder on your muscles and increases the amount of impact between your feet and your ground, which can be arduous for beginner runners. Furthermore beginner runners who increase stride length tend to compensate by lowering stride frequency, counteracting the benefit of longer strides.

You can measure you stride frequency by simply counting the number of your strides for 20 seconds and then multiply this by three to produce your stride frequency per minute. If you measure or approximate your stride length you can even estimate how far you travel in a minute.

Similarly, as a runner you need to develop an understanding between the position of your hips and your feet. When your feet are planted in front of your body you cannot push of the ground effectively. Your hips must be above or in front of your feet for you to push off the ground. Therefore a tendency to produce a long stride results in an excessive amount of time where the feet are either airborne or behind the body. Short, efficient strides are simply better until you can produce powerful, swift longer strides.

It has been suggested you can practice proper stride length and running technique through minimalist running - running with either minimalist shoes or no footwear. Of course, running across a pavement with no shoes is a bad idea, but practising across grass or soft ground for a few minutes can give you an impression of how you 'should' run. When practising this way, try to run fast or outright sprint, because this will force you to position your feet efficiently.

Another technical flaw is keeping your upper body tense whilst you run. When running there should be a natural rhythm to your upper body, with your arms being gently pumped back and forward and your shoulders accompanying them. You should also ensure that your jaw is not tensed and your back is not upright but not rigid.

If you realize that your upper body is tensed whilst you run, a method you can use to relax your body is to deliberately tense your upper body muscles for a moment. After you have tensed your muscles, the sensation of relaxing the muscles should come more naturally. Alternatively another method you can use to help your upper body relax is to lock your hands together and rest them upon your head. Locking your hands and your arms in this way ensures that your shoulders, arms and back are relaxed (or if you tense your muscles they will tire very quickly).

When running, you should also focus on ensuring that your foot strikes the floor directly beneath your knee. If your foot strikes the floor in front of you, you increase the risk of injury and place a greater level of strain on your muscles and bones. When pushing upwards you should push up from your toes rather than your heel in a spring-like motion. Your feet should never slap the floor but collide with the floor gently and smoothly in a rolling-like motion.

Similarly you should keep your elbows bent at around a 90 degree angle and below your chest. This helps ensures the efficiency of your run but also ensures that you are not tensing your muscles without realizing.

It can also help to exercise and strengthen you core muscles whilst working on your running. Strong glutes and abdominal muscles can help keep your back upright and keep your form correct without having to explicitly think about these factors whilst you run.

When running you should keep your head and your chest facing forward. When endurance running, especially when your stamina is starting to flag, it can be easily to sag downwards and let your head, neck and chest sink towards the floor.

Running Up Hills

To run up hills you should shorten your stride even more and increase the frequency of your strides to compensate. It can be tempting to lengthen your stride further but this is incredibly harsh on your muscles and your bones and joints which you connect to the sloped ground at an angle. A slight lean forward with your entire body is fine but you should be leaning forward above the waist and this will compromise your form and make it harder to run.

Also, raise your knees slightly higher than usual, using the lifting power of the thighs and glutes – you need to raise your leg higher in order to give your feet room to land. Whilst running up hills you will push up using the front and mid-sections of your feet rather than the sole but ensure that you raise your legs behind you to compensate.

Overall running up hills is great to work the glutes and hamstrings harder than usual and to think about your form in greater depth. However be careful not to overwork your calves as this might limit your ability to run normally.

Running Down Hills

Running down a hill is easier on the respiratory system and your muscles are aided by gravity instead of fighting it. Nonetheless, running down a hill challenges your legs in a unique way, forcing muscle movements and joints into positions that do not normally occur when running. Due to this it can be easy to injure yourself when running down a hill if you employ the wrong technique.

Running down a hill actually causes more muscle tear than running normal. When you run straight the muscles in your legs contract and shorten as you push of the ground. However when you run downhill your legs actually elongate and extend, creating small tears in the muscle fiber. This is a good way to challenge your calves and hamstrings if you find yourself at a growth plateau, but be aware you will feel the tiredness and fatigue in the morning.

Running down a hill at any considerable speed requires training the muscles in advance. You will need to find a hill to run down that has a gentle incline (try no more than 10% - you can use GPS and map data to help) as sharper inclines will produce higher injury rates. Likewise try to avoid running on concrete or harder surfaces; favour gravel or grass which absorb impact.

Instead of leaning back you want to keep your posture upright with a specific focus on keeping your gaze and chest facing forward. You will also want to shorten your stride and increase your cadence, using the front and midsection of your foot to absorb impact frequently, rather than harsh jarring longer strides where you use the heel to slow down.

Pacing

The trick to long distance running is pacing. If you start too fast you will exhaust your reserves of energy and run out of breath before you finish your run. You can also build up the waste products of exercise in your system faster than your body can deal with them, resulting is muscle fatigue which forces you to slow down.

Furthermore you can also deplete your muscles glycogen stores, which will cause your body to start burning fat – a process which is slower and results in an energy lag. Finally you can also raise your core temperature to a particularly high amount, causing you to sweat more than you need and exert your body to cool yourself down. However, conversely, go too slow and you will not challenge yourself enough or feel the benefits of your run.

So how do you achieve the correct pace? Well one way is to warm up before your exercise period, which helps acclimatize your body to the level of exertion it can be comfortable with. Although it might sound strange, the shorter your period of exercise is, the longer you should warm up. For large periods of running such as half-marathons and marathons, you can't afford to waste too much energy pre-workout. Furthermore your body has plenty of time to warm up during the activity itself and achieve a pleasant pace; essentially the first few miles of a marathon are your warm-up, where you start slow and gradually increase your pace.

Conversely for a shorter period of exercise you don't have to worry about wasting your glycogen stores or fatiguing your muscles. Likewise you don't have time during the running session itself to warm your body up – you need to be ready to go from the moment you start, hence the longer warm-up.

Another tip for achieving the correct pace is simply experiment. There are many different gradients and paces between a lethargic jog and a full paced sprint but we tend to only stick to these extremes. Instead you should try going for a run, starting the first mile or designated length at your lowest pace and incrementing your effort upwards by a little bit each length or mile. Using this method you will soon start to understand your body and the difference between a gentle pace, a comfortable but challenging pace, an unsustainable pace, a fast pace and so on.

In addition to experimenting, another way to keep your pace in check is to be mindful of your body as you run. To a certain extent 'zoning out' is how many people cope with the mental aspect of running – ignoring the pain and uncomfortable sensations in their body by thinking about something else or listening to music.

However when you are distracted you are not moderating your body and your pace. You need to frequently ask yourself if your breathing is too fast or too slow, if your muscles feel tired, if your form is correct and so on. By constantly staying on track with how you want to pace yourself, you prevent yourself from burning out or going too slow simply due to not being aware.

Chapter 4 – Mentality

Although you can learn all the technical details of running at the end of the day the most important factor in whether your running is successful and how fast your running practice grows, is your own mind. You need to train yourself to perform and push on once your body starts telling you that it wants to quit.

There are various ways you can alter your thinking to give your spirit a bit more bite. First you can focus on the positives of a situation rather than the negatives. This little piece of advice sounds redundant when talking about running, but it is in fact ubiquitous. For example, instead of becoming down when it is raining and cold outside, be grateful for the days when it is warm and breezy. Instead of being irritated when you are injured or aching, appreciate all the times your muscles and body are feeling energized.

Likewise recognize that you have the ability to control your thoughts – you don't have to let negative thoughts pester you and bring you down. Start a positive thinking habit by just being aware of when you are thinking negatively. Then when you recognize a negative thought, consider a more positive alternative.

You don't have to deny the existence of a problem or brainwash yourself and see the world through rose-tinted glasses, but you can think in terms of solutions and redeeming qualities. At the very least instead of focusing on what is wrong you can simply direct your attention to something different as a momentary distraction. In the case of running, this can often be the music you are listening to or the environment that you run past.

As a side note on injuries, instead of seeing them purely as problems, try to interpret them as obstacles. This is more than trite life-coach advice; if you are consistently getting injured you're doing something wrong and you are not listening to your body. It's one thing to push your body when it starts to feel like it's getting tired – it's another thing to ignore that ankle or knee joint that is starting to hurt. Use your injuries as wake-up signs to the signals that you are missing.

If you ever find that you are bored of your training or simply unenthusiastic, try shaking up your routine or simply doing something different. Your body adapts to the routine you perform, resulting in less challenge and less difficulty as you repeat those motions. Doing something different forces your body to face a new challenge with the prospect of a new reward.

Never perceive your running habit as a chore. The moment you start to think of running as a duty or a chore it will become a burden. Instead re-iterate to yourself the reasons why you are running and try to feel excited for those reasons. Weight loss, energy, fitness, strength, and the famous runners high. It doesn't matter what your reasons are but you should feel good when you think about them.

Although you might be training for a better body image, you also need to learn to put away your self-esteem too. There's nothing wrong with being motivated by the promise of a beach body but if you are too invested in how you look, you will be deterred whenever your progress stalls or doesn't progress at the speed at which you want.

You will reach temporary plateaus and even setbacks as you continue to train and you need to have the calmness and tranquility of mind to keep your cool.

Setting goals has been proven to improve gains and performance in athletics and other areas of performance. Nonetheless when using goals it's important to establish and work with them in the correct way, else you may discourage yourself and fall into negative thinking habits. Good goals follow the S.M.A.R.T criteria, which stands for:

Specific
Measurable
Attainable
Relevant
Time Orientated

These qualities are relatively straight forward. The specific goal entails that your goal is well-defined and detailed – instead of just 'be fitter' or 'start running', a specific goal might be 'run twice a week every week for 2 months'. A measurable goal is a goal that can be easily measured – the goal of just being 'fitter' is too vague to be evaluated, but the goal of running a 4 minute mile can be measured for success.

An attainable goal is a goal that is realistically achievable. If you are obese setting a goal of running a sub-4 minute mile in 1 month may not be physically or mentally possible. Establishing a goal of a sub-4 minute mile in just 18 months? Feasible.

Relevant goals are goals that are relevant to your overall desires – if your goal is a 4 minute mile, setting a goal about saving money isn't helpful (as you might expect).

Finally the time-bound criterion is that your goals should have a time limit. With no deadline on your goals it is easy to procrastinate and delay, but knowing that you have a goal for this week or this month forces you to act *now*.

In addition to the smart criteria your goals should also be malleable. As previously touched upon, sometimes you will reach temporary plateaus, sometimes you will get injured, have setbacks or even suffer from a lapse of motivation. Regardless if you get too disheartened by not reaching your exact goal, you will struggle to achieve. It is better to aim high and fall short than not to aim at all.

When running for performance you also need to banish doubts. If you are attempting to set a new personal record or take a challenge you've never attempted, doubt can gnaw at you before you run and as you run, distracting you from your task.

You need to have confidence in your abilities, or at the very least, take your mind away from the doubt your feel. Rationalize to yourself why you can achieve your task, such as considering your recent or comparable achievements. Alternatively seek social support, voicing your concerns to other people who share your interests and can alleviate that pressure you feel.

You also need to avoid comparing yourself to others, especially when your running is more of a hobby than a career. There will always be a bigger fish or someone who is better in some regard. If you endlessly compare yourself to others you are probably going to find that you come up short, ruining your self-confidence in the process. Instead focus on what you can control – your own actions and your own feelings.

Chapter 5 – Stay Safe, Fit, and Healthy

When running safety should always be a concern. If you are not careful it is easy to be hit a vehicle that's not paying adequate attention or place yourself in a vulnerable position. Therefore there a few tips you should always adhere to whenever you run.

Firstly, tell someone that you are going out so they know to be suspicious if you do not return. Better still, try to run with another person or join a running group so you have safety in numbers. Some people also enjoy running with a dog, yet if you are fit and running long distances a dog can actually struggle to match the running endurance of a human.

Always run with at least a mobile phone so you can contact someone in case of an emergency – this might include getting help for yourself, but also for someone who you encounter who is in trouble. If possible it's also best if you carry ID with you so that if you do encounter trouble and fall unconscious people can identify you and locate emergency contacts. Many runners also attach medical information to an item that they bring with them on a run, or write it on the inside of their shoes.

It is also wise to carry some cash with you just in case you need to ring a taxi or take public transport back home instead of walking or running or need to buy anything in emergency.

Always presume that cars can't see you and take personal responsibility for your visibility, wearing high-visibility and reflective gear when running along roadsides. If running in the dark, invest in a head light or another lighting option. It may feel awkward, but safe and awkward is better than comfortable and dangerous. It is best to avoid running during the night altogether, if possible. At the very least if you are running during the night, stick to public and well-lit places; never run down an alley or deserted street by yourself.

When running down a road, run facing towards the traffic, instead of having it behind you, which enables you to see if a car is possibly going to collide with you. Drivers generally have an easier time seeing you if you are facing them as well.

Avoid listening to music whilst running, especially if you do run anywhere where vehicles are nearby. Jamming to the newest beat isn't worth being hit by a bus that you couldn't hear approaching. If you must listen to music whilst you run in a public place, only keep a single headphone in your ear at a reasonable volume so you can stay aware of surrounding noise.

Be careful when running early in the morning and late in the evening. People can be tired and cranky at this time, making their driving worse. Also be aware of the potential danger that other people may present and avoid groups of people and isolated places where you may be vulnerable. Use your own gut instinct here – if you feel like something is wrong, just take a different route or double-back and return later.

Make yourself clear to any people that you may encounter as you run. People are notoriously spatially oblivious to runners and you shouldn't expect them to move out the way of you – call out ahead of you to make sure people get out of your way, especially down narrow paths.

Avoid antagonizing or responding to any verbal harassment. Some people, for some unknown reason, find it hilarious to laugh at struggling runners, catcall or perform some other idiotic provocation. Just ignore them and keep running – there is no need to turn a minor problem into a bigger issue.

If you are strongly concerned about your safety, you can use tracking devices which friends and family can link to in order to know your location as you run. You can even alter your route to make it harder for people to know your running patterns and anticipate your behaviour if you fear that you may be being stalked or followed.

Some people also feel the need to carry mace or pepper spray with them in order to deal with any potential attackers – it can never hurt to be prepared, especially if you are particularly vulnerable or you know you are running through a high risk area. Alternatively some runners also take it upon themselves to learn basic self defence in order to fend off attackers as well as carry a noise alert or distress siren in order to gather help.

Of course in most circumstances this level of preparation will be somewhat excessive but go as far with your self-defence as you feel necessary; some neighborhoods are more dangerous than others.

Dealing with Immediate Injury

In the previous chapters various methods of injury prevention were outlined. However knowing how to deal with an injury that occurs whilst running is also important.

Firstly, it's important to make a distinction between immediate and sharp pain and mild pain or aches that slowly grow and escalate over time. The latter suggests that there is some problem caused by poor form or weakness that is getting worse. This needs to be dealt with, but you can complete your run first then research what you are doing wrong later.

A rapid on-set, immediate and severe pain suggests something is heavily wrong and that you should probably stop immediately. If you have difficulty breathing and aching in your chest, be mindful of any sensations of faintness, extreme sweating or aching in the neck and shoulders, as these might indicate problems with your lungs or heart. If the problem subsides within a few minutes you are probably ok, but it is best to check up with your GP nonetheless.

Watch out for severe incremental pain in the foot which eventually becomes unbearable. This may be caused by a stress fracture, where the bones in the foot fracture and can no longer bear weight. Stop running immediately and seek treatment.

Also never continue to run if you have swollen your ankle, especially if swelling and redness has occurred. You may be able to tough it out and complete your run, but continued activity will damage your ankle more and cause you to take longer to recovery.

Hay Fever

Hay fever can play havoc with a runner's ability to run long distances and enjoy their runs, but with a few simple steps the condition can be mostly alleviated. Hay fever is caused by your own body's immune system reacting to pollen, resulting in inflammation and soreness in the sinuses, eyes and throat.

Pollen can be separated into three large categories; tree pollen, grass pollen and weed pollen. These tree types of pollen are released during different times of the year with tree pollen typically being released in spring to the beginning of summer, grass pollen is released from the end of the spring to the start of summer and weed pollen is mostly released during late autumn.

If you suspect that you are suffering from hay fever understanding what type of hay fever you are suffering can help you be prepared to cope with your symptoms. Hay fever is more prevalent in people who are related to other people who suffer from hay fever, asthma or eczema.

Above and beyond annoyance and irritation, hay fever poses a legitimate obstacle to running performance as it can drastically block your nasal capacity, reducing the amount of oxygen that can enter your lungs. It can result in your body becoming tired due to your immune system fighting an invisible threat and sap your concentration, affecting your technique.

To reduce the impact of hay fever there are several options. Air pollution can exacerbate the impact of hay fever, so trying to run away from urban places and roadsides where air pollution is prevalent can help. However avoiding places with lots of vegetation and pollen sources is also wise, so you can either try to run indoors or find an open place that lacks fauna growth.

Wearing sunglass can help limit your eyes exposure to pollen, although this can be somewhat impractical and difficult during the run. You can also avoid running during the time of the day where plants pollinate – early morning or late afternoon. If you are fortunate to have a flexible schedule, this means either running during the middle of the day or waiting until the evening. Some people even resort to taking their running gear with them to the office and going for a run during their lunch break.

After you have run ensure that you wash and clean your clothes regularly, as during the pollination season pollen will settle on your clothes, causing an allergic response sooner the next time you wear those clothes. In a similar manner avoid airing or hanging your post-workout clothes indoors as this will just spread the pollen inside.

In terms of diet, making an effort to consume a high amount of vitamin A can help keep the lining inside your respiratory system working effectively, reducing the build up of allergic effects. Vitamin A is particularly prominent in liver, sweet potato and fresh vegetables, including spinach.

Vitamin B5 is also known to be influential in allergic reactions and can be found in most meats and eggs. It can also be found in peanut butter. Other dietary supplements or requirements to manage allergic reactions and hay fever can include zinc, found in bran, poultry, red meat and shellfish as well as numerous fortified products. Likewise magnesium is also beneficial and can be found in a wide variety of foods, including leafy greens, nuts, seeds, fish, dark chocolate and some whole grains.

Ultimately if you eat a nutritious and well-balanced diet you shouldn't need supplementation to consume enough vitamins and minerals. However if you do want to go the extra mile, cod liver oil contains a high amount of vitamin A and may be able to help.

In addition to taking anti-histamines and eye drops to help solve hay fever, you can also try buying some locally made honey. Local honey will be produced from bees that collect pollen from local plants, therefore containing some of the chemical compounds that are triggering your allergic reactions. This isn't a bad thing however – it is though that by ingesting these compounds through eating honey you can develop a tolerance to local pollen, as if the honey were a vaccine.

For people who suffer severely with hay fever seek medical advice from your GP or pharmacist. It is important to be as proactive as possible as therapeutic solutions to hay fever are typically most effective when treatment starts before the pollination season.

Asthma

Running also poses significant problems to people who suffer from asthma. However don't let any initial difficulties you face deter you, as exercise is beneficial to people with asthma. In fact exercise is great for asthma, as it boosts the efficiency of the lungs, bolsters the immune system and therefore reduces susceptibility to colds and coughs, promotes weight loss which is a contributor to asthma symptoms and improves mood, which can also worsen asthma symptoms.

Furthermore asthma doesn't have to limit athletic performance with many athletes and people in physically demanding jobs having asthma themselves. The key is managing your asthma symptoms well. If your asthma is particularly severe currently and your fitness levels are lacking, it may be wise to use a gentler form of exercise to improve your condition first. Avoiding areas which are heavy with air pollution is also wise for people with asthma, so avoid roadsides with petrol fumes and areas with high pollen counts of freshly cut grass.

It can also be beneficial to construct your runs in a particular way by having recovery sessions in the midst of your running. Some people can suffer from exercise induced asthma when their body is under particularly high stress and they need to breathe especially deeply to supply their body with oxygen. Allowing your body to calm down and for your breathing to become deep and slow will ensure you do not put yourself in a position where an asthma attack can occur.

Likewise you can also avoid training for speed and timing and focus on long distance running. Speed running generally is more exerting and more likely to trigger an asthma attack.

Taking a bottle of water with you can help keep your airways from becoming too dry, which can leads to coughs and soreness. However cold water can also tickle your throat, so taking lukewarm or warm water is best, especially on colder days. Warming up can help your body adjust and your core temperature to rise, helping you deal with cold air better, so don't try to skip it.

Furthermore it's also important to cover up any time the air is cold. Most people make the mistake of just trying to cover up their chest and torso without covering their mouth and nostrils to prevent sharp cold air from directly penetrating their lungs. Purchase a light face mask specifically designed for exercise in order to receive enough air.

Also, inform your friends and family that you are going for a run before you leave, so they are aware if you get into trouble and do not return. Above all other advice, ensure that you always bring your inhalers with you so if an asthma attack does occur, you are prepared.

Conclusion

Running is one of the best ways you can improve your health but it can also a rewarding and invigorating hobby that can improve your mood and outlook.

It's no coincidence that the streets, roads, and local parks are full of joggers. The post runs endorphin release creates a feeling that leaves many runners wanting to get more. It really can be an addictive hobby. However this is one addiction that will serve you well!

So what are you waiting for, get out there and join the millions who are already running and feeling better every day.

By having read this guide you should now be ready to kick-start a new running resolution or if you already run, take your hobby to the next level. Good luck!

www.ingramcontent.com/pod-product-compliance
Lightning Source LLC
Chambersburg PA
CBHW071127280526
45787CB00003B/1206